I0449781

How to Buy a Water Filter

Everything you need to know to select the right home water filter for you and your family.

By: Stefan Roots

http://www.dirtywaterdude.com/

HOW TO BUY A WATER FILTER. EVERYTHING YOU NEED TO KNOW ABOUT WATER FILTERS TO OBTAIN CLEAN, SAFE DRINKING WATER AT HOME.

COPYRIGHT © 2017 Stefan Roots

ISBN-13   978-1548275990

ISBN-10   1548275999

Printed in the United States of America.

Table of Contents

1. About the Dirty Water Dude

In the early 1980s I married a lady from Georgia who hated the taste of the water in Philadelphia. She learned of a place we could get water for free from an outdoor free flowing spring. For months, we joined others and brought home bottles of water from that spring.

One day a guy pulled off to the side of the road like he was coming for some spring water. He walked up to the dispenser without any bottles so we knew he had another objective. He told us the water we were getting wasn't clean even though there was a sign right there that said the water was tested monthly.

At first we blew him off like he was a crazy man until he said, "You know deer run all around in those hills. There's no doubt that there's deer piss in the water you're drinking."

That was the last day we got water from that spring.

Later that year we invested in water filter purchased from a company we both trusted. Neither of us knew anything about what the filter was designed to filter, but we both agreed our water tasted a lot better.

We maintained that filter through our short marriage and she held on to it for many years. I never owned a water filter again until 2013.

Like most people, I never trusted tap water to be as safe as bottled water for drinking until I stumbled into a career with a waste water treatment company. I earned a certificate at the local community college for waste water treatment and passed the state certification tests. My background in engineering made me curious about the process of drinking water treatment. I read everything I could on the Safe Drinking Water laws and kept up on current news regarding water issues from across America.

And then Flint happened.

As tragic as Flint, Michigan became, I knew there were similar – and even worse – tragedies going on across the country with drinking water. I became upset at the media coverage of Flint because I felt it created more fear and finger pointing than it offered solutions. Even today when I talk to people, they have little knowledge of what happened in Flint other than the water was polluted with lead.

That's when I decided to create a company to help others understand the issues regarding drinking water and advocate for preaching on how important it is to obtain a certified water filter so people can receive clean safe drinking water at home.

2. Mission Statement

The mission of my company - Dirty Water Dude - is to help educate on the issues concerning drinking water and introduce the best available solution to obtain clean safe drinking water at home.

Let me break down that key phrases in that mission statement.

EDUCATE...

DirtyWaterDude.com is a site that is constantly updated with a host of recent articles, podcasts episodes, videos, and forums that address all aspects of drinking water to aid in learning what's going on with water from across the country.

...ISSUES CONCERNING DRINKNG WATER...

The issues with drinking water span many areas: Federal and local government regulations; municipal water treatment systems; infrastructure including water mains and service lines; source water including rivers, lakes, and streams; waste water treatment; known contaminants not being treated; the media; and public perception.

…THE BEST AVAILABLE SOLUTIONS…

There is plenty of room for improvement in federal and local government regulations; new technologies in municipal water treatment systems; replacement of aging water mains and lead based service lines; eliminating known contaminants from the water; better media coverage of water issues; and more education so people will have an accurate perception of the real problems with their drinking water.

…OBTAIN CLEAN SAFE DRINKING WATER FROM HOME

A certified water filter is your last line of defense to obtain clean safe drinking water at home. The best filters are certified to be assured to remove the contaminants they are rated to remove. Not all home water filters are the same which is why it's critical that you identify which contaminants you need to eliminate and install the proper filter certified to remove those contaminants.

3. Bottled Water versus Tap Water

In 2016, bottled water outsold bottled soda for the first time ever, and the trend is likely to continue.

Most people believe bottled water is better than tap water. Some folks never drink tap water and only drink bottled water at home and when they are away from home. Whenever there is an issue with the municipal water system the authorities always provide bottle water to their customers while they fix the problem. Bottled water is definitely the most convenient way to consume water when you are away from other sources of drinking water.

Municipal water systems claim their water (tap water) is safer to drink because they must comply with stringent federal Environmental Protection Agency (EPA) regulations to stay in business. Bottled water is regulated by the Food and Drug Administration (FDA) which is considered less stringent than the EPA.

Bottled water also has the issue that the plastic bottles may cause a health concern and the plastic bottles definitely cause an environmental concern with their disposal.

The cost of bottle water far exceeds the cost of drinking water from the tap. For $1 you can buy a 16 oz bottle of water. That same $1 will buy you 500-16oz glasses of tap water. So, you can get a drink of water for $1 or get 500 drinks of water for the same $1.

The goal of most bottled water companies is to provide a product that taste better than tap water. By removing chlorine, bottled water tastes and smells better to most people. Bottled water also removes dirt and scale that generally gives it a consistently clear appearance which can't be said for tap water at all times.

Many bottled water companies purchase municipal water and run it through filters. In many instances, bottled water is the same water you can make from your tap if you installed a basic water filter.

There aren't many bottles of water with a 'Born On Date' stamped on it like that beer company does. You never know when the water was bottled, how long it sat in a warehouse, on a truck, in the sun, or on a store shelf. That could be a problem because water doesn't like to sit still. The longer it sits, the more potential for harm.

As an experiment, sit a bottle of unopened water outside in the sunlight. Come back a week later and unscrew the cap. Chances are it has changed in appearance and gained an odor.

Tap water is at its best when it leaves the municipal water system, but then it must travel through pipes to get to your home. The water company is responsible for assuring the quality of the water is consistent throughout the entire distribution system, but their responsibility ends with that pipe in your street (water main). You own the pipe that brings water from the water main to your home (service line). Unless they are checking every faucet in every home, there's no way to be sure of the water quality that comes into your home.

There is no denying that both bottled water and tap water contain contaminants. Many contaminants can be eliminated from tap water with a certified water filter in the home. Unfortunately, the only home filter for bottled water is a pitcher/carafe filter and most of them aren't certified to remove anything more than what most bottled water has already been filtered for – chlorine and particulates. You must read the product performance sheets to find the few pitcher water filters that are certified to remove health related contaminants. (Keep reading. I teach you how to do that in later chapters).

The one main advantage of bottled water is convenience. Other than that, it could be just as contaminated as tap water, if not more so.

4. How a Water Filter Works

Most home filters are made of activated carbon that is compressed into a block and is often wrapped with a fabric like substance.

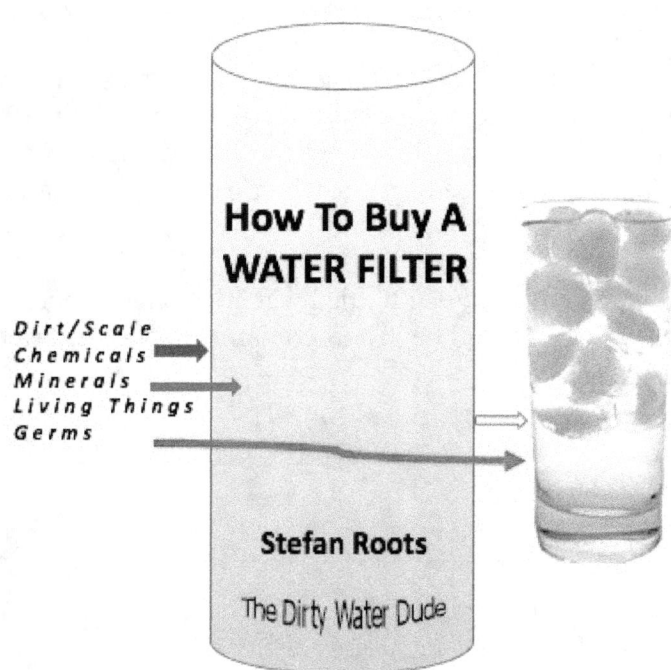

When the water enters the filter housing, the very large particles are trapped by the fabric (the top arrow). That's why the surface of the filter is brown when it's time to be replaced. Water then passes through the fabric and the small carbon material is packed so closely together that it traps smaller particles within the filter block (the middle arrow).

Activated carbon is a process that puts a magnetic charge on the carbon and many of the contaminates are of an opposite magnetic charge which break from the water molecule and attaches to the carbon filter (adsorption).

Unfortunately, carbon doesn't trap everything. Some metals and most living organisms, among other things, pass right through (bottom arrow).

In the end, the water that exits a filter has considerably less dirt, scale, and contaminants.

Water filters are rated to work for only so many gallons of water passing through it. Once you've exceeded that volume, the contaminants trapped in the filter reduce the effectiveness of the filter because there is no more room for contaminants to be stored in the filter. To use a filter beyond its rated life could produce water even worse than the contaminated water that goes into it.

Because of this fact, filter cartridges must be replaced when they reach their rated life. The smaller the filter, the more frequently it needs to be replaced. On average, you will spend

$100 a year on filter cartridge replacements regardless of the type of filter unit you buy. Of course, the filter housing is not affected by this so you don't have to trash the whole unit and get a new one. All you need to do is replace the filter cartridge when they reach their gallon limit or time limit.

An example of a filter life expectancy listing:

'Good for 300 gallons or 6 months.'

5. Different Types of Water Filters

Although there are hundreds of brands of home water filters, they all rely on a small number of technologies to remove contaminants. That does not mean that every filter that uses a given technology is as good as another, but it does mean that you can get a good idea of the general pros and cons of the different systems relatively easily.

Besides the varied technologies, there are only 7 physical types of filter units.

Here are the typical filter unit types:

Pitcher or Carafe

A water filter pitcher is filled with tap water (or bottled water) and is filtered when water is poured into the pitcher over an activated carbon filter. The filter generally only reduces chlorine and particulates (NSF 42) but some go a step further and remove lead and mercury. Because the filters are very small, they need to be replaced frequently. The replacement filters are normally sold in packs of three or more because they are small and need to be replaced after approximately 40 gallons of use. Most filtered water pitchers are just shy of 1 gallon in size and easily fit in a refrigerator.

Faucet Mounted

This filter attaches to the end of your water faucet. By default, water flows straight through the faucet for tasks like washing dishes, washing your hands, or filling a bucket. When you want drinking water, pull a stem on the attached filter unit and the water passes through the filter and into your glass.

These filters are certified as NSF 42 and NSF 53. It's important to understand the NSA Certification standards and the unit's performance specification when buying a faucet mounted filter. Also, filter units come with or without a filter life indicator to alert you when the filter needs to be replaced.

Because the filters on faucet mounted units are small, they need to be replaced more frequently than filters for a countertop or under-sink filter unit.

Usually, the flow through the filter slows down when the filter is clogged. This could occur sooner than the manufacturer recommends replacement if your water is much dirtier than normal.

These units do not mount on all faucet styles, especially the more modern types.

Counter Top

These units work similarly to the faucet mounted units. The filter unit sits on the counter and tubing from the unit is attached to the end of the faucet. When the stem is pulled, water is diverted from the faucet through tubing to the filter unit and filtered water exits the unit and travels through a different tube that dispenses at the faucet connection.

Another type of counter top unit uses an auxiliary spout to dispense the filtered water. Tubing still connects from the unit to the end of the faucet but there is no return tube to the faucet. Instead, the filtered water is dispensed though the auxiliary spout. This arrangement may require skills to install and plumb.

Counter top units use a range of technologies including activated carbon, reverse osmosis and ultraviolet light. They come with or without a filter life indicator to alert you when the filter needs to be replaced.

Because these units are much larger than the faucet mounted units, the filters generally last much longer before cartridges need to be replaced.

Under Sink

This is an identical unit as the counter top unit but it doesn't attach to the faucet. The filter unit sits below the sink next to the cold water line. Hardware pokes a hole in the cold water line and sends the water through the filter. The water is dispensed through an auxiliary dispenser that normally screws right into the counter top or at the sink if you have access to a spare 'punch out' that is usually reserved for a trigger sprayer. When you want filtered water, you push the lever on the auxiliary dispenser and fill your glass allowing you to use your faucet and receive filtered water at the same time since nothing attaches directly to your faucet.

Under sink units use a range of technologies including activated carbon, reverse osmosis and ultra violet light. They come with or without a filter life indicator to alert you when the filter needs to be replaced.

These units are attractive if you don't have a lot of counter top space or if you prefer to hide your filter unit behind the cabinet doors. They almost always require installation and plumbing skills.

Refrigerator

Most new refrigerators with a water and ice dispenser include a water filter located inside the refrigerator. These filters are small and need to be replaced frequently. The refrigerator will come with or without a filter life indicator to alert you when the filter needs to be replaced.

Some counter top and below counter filter units can bypass the small refrigerator filter and be rigged to filter the water that enters the refrigerator. This will likely require some plumbing skills.

Refrigerator filter units normally use activated carbon and can include ultraviolet light if you rig up a counter top unit that employs that technology.

Whole House

Whole house filters come in a variety of configurations. Since most people are only concerned about improving their drinking water, I don't focus on whole house filters. They are preferred by homes that are served with well water.

Whole house filters can cost around $5000 to install and because all the water coming into the home is flowing through the filter unit, the filter replacement costs can be expensive.

Whole House filter units have the best ability to be configured to use every technology available and many whole house filters combine technologies to achieve a desired contaminant reduction. They come with or without a filter life indicator to alert you when the filter needs to be replaced.

You must consider if it's worth the extra costs to have filtered drinking water and filtered toilet water, filtered shower water, filtered water for your grass, filtered water to wash your clothes, and filtered water to wash your car. That's what you get with a whole house water filter.

Shower Filter

A shower filter screws into the shower head to remove chlorine and dirt from the water. Chlorine in hot steamy environments have been known to create a mist that may contains a cancer causing agent.

6. Types of Water Filter Technologies

The Environmental Working Group does an excellent job of defining the various technologies used to filter water. The majority of home water filter units (Point of Use) are set in the kitchen and attach to the end of a faucet or the cold water line under the sink. Whole house water filters (Point of Entry) connect in the basement of most homes where the water line comes into the structure.

Activated carbon block is the most common filter technology found in filters certified as NSF 42&53. However, these filters lack the ability to effectively remove common "inorganic" pollutants.

Reverse osmosis filters (NSF 58) do a great job of effectively removing common "inorganic" pollutants but don't remove chlorine, trihalomethanes or volatile organic chemicals (VOCs) which activated carbon does a great job removing.

Ultraviolet light (NSF 55) is the only non-chemical technology to kill bacteria and other microorganisms.

Here is a great collection of the different water filter technology definitions:

From http://www.ewg.org/research/ewgs-water-filter-buying-guide/filter-technology

Carbon/Activated Carbon: Activated carbon chemically bonds
with and removes some contaminants in water filtered through
it. Carbon filters vary greatly in effectiveness: Some just
remove chlorine and improve taste and odor, while others
remove a wide range of contaminants including asbestos, lead,
mercury and volatile organic compounds (VOCs). However,
activated carbon cannot effectively remove common
"inorganic" pollutants such as arsenic, fluoride, hexavalent
chromium, nitrate and perchlorate. Generally, carbon filters
come in two forms, carbon block and granulated activated
carbon.

Carbon Block: Carbon block filters contain pulverized
activated carbon that is shaped into blocks under high
pressure. They are typically more effective than granulated
activated carbon filters because they have more surface area.
Their effectiveness depends in part on how quickly water
flows through.

Granulated Activated Carbon: These filters contain fine grains
of activated carbon. They are typically less effective than
carbon block filters because they have a smaller surface area
of activated carbon. Their effectiveness also depends on how
quickly water flows through.

Reverse Osmosis: This process pushes water through a semi-
permeable membrane that blocks particles larger than water
molecules. Reverse osmosis can remove many contaminants
not removed by activated carbon, including arsenic, fluoride,
hexavalent chromium, nitrates and perchlorate. However,
reverse osmosis does not remove chlorine, trihalomethanes or

volatile organic chemicals (VOCs). Many reverse osmosis systems include an activated carbon component than can remove these other contaminants. Quality can vary tremendously in both the membrane system and the carbon filter typically used with it. Consumers should also be aware that reverse osmosis filters use 3-to-20 times more water than they produce. Because they waste quite a bit of water, they are best used for drinking and cooking water only.

UV (ultraviolet): These systems use ultraviolet light to kill bacteria and other microorganisms. They cannot remove chemical contaminants.

Ceramic: Ceramic filters have very small holes throughout the material that block solid contaminants such as cysts and sediments. They do not remove chemical contaminants.

Deionization: These filters use an ion exchange process that removes mineral salts and other electrically charged molecules (ions) from water. The process cannot remove non-ionic contaminants (including trihalomethanes and other common volatile organic compounds) or microorganisms.

Distillation: This technology heats water enough to vaporize it and then condenses the steam back into water. The process removes minerals, many bacteria and viruses and chemicals that have a higher boiling point than water. It cannot remove chlorine, trihalomethanes or volatile organic chemicals (VOCs).

Fibredyne block: This is a proprietary type of carbon block filter that claims to have a higher sediment holding capacity than other carbon block filters.

Ion Exchange: This technology passes water over a resin that replaces undesirable ions with others that are more desirable. One common application is water softening, which replaces calcium and magnesium with sodium. The resin must be periodically "recharged" with replacement ions.

Mechanical Filters: Like ceramic filters, these filters are riddled with small holes that remove contaminants such as cysts and sediments. They are often used in conjunction with other kinds of technologies, but sometimes are used alone. They cannot remove chemical contaminants.

Ozone: Ozone kills bacteria and other microorganisms and is often used in conjunction with other filtering technologies. It is not effective in removing chemical contaminants.

Water Softeners: These devices typically use an ion exchange process to lower levels of calcium and magnesium (which can build up in plumbing and fixtures) as well barium and certain forms of radium. They do not remove most other contaminants. Since water softeners usually replace calcium and magnesium with sodium, treated water typically has high sodium content. Some people may be advised by their physicians to avoid softened water. For the same reason, it is also not recommended for watering plants and gardens.

7. What is NSF Certification?

While no federal regulations exist for residential water treatment devices, several voluntary national standards establish minimum requirements for the safety and performance of products used to treat home drinking water.

Founded in 1944, NSF International is a US based, independent, accredited organization, whose mission is to protect and improve global human health through the development of standards and testing/certification for a wide range of products and systems. Certification to an NSF standard ensures that your product meets the regulatory requirements for the U.S., and can often meet or fulfill the testing requirements for many other countries as well.

Market leaders strive to attain NSF certification as a mark of distinction that assures their customers that their product is safe for use and can effectively remove contaminants in drinking water. (From NSF.org)

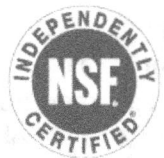

NSF International is a global public health organization that certifies the performance claims of companies that manufacture almost anything that has anything to do with food (water is considered food). This includes appliances, chemicals, equipment, containers, and more.

NSF is considered the official certifier of home water filters units and their filter cartridges.

Typically, a water filter manufacturer designs and builds their filter to remove contaminants to a certain level. For example, they may claim to reduce chlorine by 90% and lead by 97%. Many people are suspicious when a manufacturer makes those types of claims?

To remove all doubt, a water filter manufacturer submits their filter to NSF to confirm that the contaminant removal they claim will be achieved at NSF labs. NSF tests the unit and if they meet or exceed the manufacturers claims, NSF allows the manufacturer to add 'NSF Certified' on the product.

NSF certification for water filters falls into several categories. NSF also identifies the contaminants they want to see reduced and to what level of reduction.

For example, NSF may state that a filter must remove at least 50% of the chlorine from the tap water passing through it. A manufacturer would have to at least meet that standard before bringing their unit to NSF for testing.

For certification purposes, the manufacturer may claim to remove 90% of chlorine and prints that on their filter performance specification sheet. If NSF tests determines the filter removed only 80% of the chlorine, NSF will not certify the filter because the manufacturer made a false claim by stating it would remove 90% of the chlorine. The unit could still be sold, but without the NSF certification logo.

However, if the NSF tests finds that the filter removes 90% or more of the chlorine, NSF gives the unit a passing grade. The manufacturer can continue to list a 90% removal because NSF found that it met or exceeded the 90% removal claim.

Practically all major water filter manufacturers certify their products with NSF. If you see a filter that doesn't have the NSF logo, I recommend you do not buy it. You're likely to find these filters sold by mail order, TV infomercials, and home shopping TV shows.

Some filters will claim that they meet NSF specifications, but they don't have the NSF logo on their unit, packaging or literature. Legally, the NSF logo can only go on a product that has been NSF approved.

Here is a real example of a filter manufacturer performance specification that claims to meet NSF standards but did not have their unit certified with NSF...

> *The Clear2O ® ADVANCED CWF500 series filter has been independently tested on over 200 contaminants to achieve water industry standards NSF/ANSI 42 and*

NSF/ANSI 53 for reduction of Chlorine, Heavy Metals, Cysts, VOC, & Other contaminants. The Clear2O® ADVANCED filter system surpasses NSF/ANSI 53 and NSF/ANSI 401 test standards for removal of Herbicides, Pesticides, Pharmaceuticals, Industrial Wastes, and PFOA's (Perfluorooctanoic Acids), man-made chemicals used in various manufacturing processes, and has been shown to be a health concern as it has been shown to be widely present in the environment and remain in the human body for long periods of time.

This unit is not NSF certified and legally cannot display the NSF logo. However, they claim to have surpassed NSF test standards.

It's up to you to believe their claim or not. If the Clear2O unit sent their unit to NSF to obtain NSF certification, there would be no doubt that their claims are verified.

NSF has a website with all the units they have approved. Sometimes it's a little tricky to find the unit you're looking for because so many companies sell products under different names than the corporate name listed on the NSF site. But, most major manufacturers retain consistent branding.

NSF listing for certified filters:
http://info.nsf.org/Certified/PwsComponents

The NSF standards are generally divided according to the product's technology. The numbers assigned to each standard reflect the order in which the standards were developed. Below are the standards and the type of technology each covers, along with a description of the purpose or intended function of the technology.

Unfortunately, I lost track of the website where the information below came from, but it's a great overview of the NSF/ANSI numbering system for their standards (or protocols) for residential water treatment devices. Notice how the NSF standards are based on the water filter technology employed.

Adsorption/Filtration (NSF/ANSI 42 & 53)

This process occurs when liquid, gas or dissolved or suspended matter adheres to the surface of, or in the pores of, an adsorbent media. Carbon filters are an example of this type of product.

Ultraviolet Treatment (NSF/ANSI 55)

These systems use ultraviolet light to disinfect water (Class A systems) or to reduce the amount of non-disease causing bacteria in water (Class B).

Treatment Systems for Emerging Contaminants (NSF/ANSI 401)

Systems covered by this standard include several types of point-of-use (POU) and point-of-entry (POE) systems that have been verified to reduce up to 15 emerging contaminants from drinking water.

Shower Filters (NSF/ANSI 177)
These products attach directly to the pipe just in front of the homeowner's showerhead.

Reverse Osmosis (NSF/ANSI 58)
These systems incorporate a process that uses reverse pressure to force water through a semi-permeable membrane. Most reverse osmosis systems incorporate one or more additional filters on either side of the membrane.

Softeners (NSF/ANSI 44)
These systems incorporate a cation exchange resin that is regenerated with sodium or potassium chloride. The softener reduces calcium and magnesium ions and replaces them with sodium or potassium ions.

Distillers (NSF/ANSI 62)
These systems heat water to the boiling point, and then collect the water vapor as it condenses, leaving behind contaminants such as heavy metals. Some contaminants that convert readily into gases, such as volatile organic chemicals, can carry over with the water vapor.

Keep in mind that certification to an NSF/ANSI standard does not mean that a product will effectively reduce all possible contaminants. It's important to verify that the product is certified under that standard for reduction of the specific impurities of most concern to you or your family.

The final paragraph is very important. It's best explained with an example.

If you are purchasing a water filter rated NSF 53, it isn't required to effectively reduce all possible contaminants that fall under NSF 53. It only has to reduce the impurity it claims to reduce. Therefore, it's important to verify from the product performance data sheet (specifications) that specific impurity you are concerned about is listed.

For example, that NSF 53 filter you're looking to buy may reduce lead by 90%. But, you are seeking a filter that also removes Mercury. Although lead and mercury are both covered under NSF 53, if the manufacturer doesn't state that it reduces Mercury on its specification sheet, the filter is still an approved NSF 53 product because it reduces lead even though it doesn't treat for Mercury.

In other words, a filter does not have to reduce every impurity that falls under a NSF standard to be approved.

NSF standards do span filter unit technologies. For example, VOCs and arsenic are health related contaminants covered under NSF 53. But a carbon based filter cannot remove arsenic. A reverse osmosis filter cannot remove VOCs. Yet, both filters can carry the NSF 53 standard if they can reduce any health related impurity listed under NSF 53.

Because of that, many filters utilize more than one technology and are certified under two or more standards. The most common combination is a NSF 42/53 filter. It removes chlorine and particulates under NSF 42, and it removes the listed health related contaminant under NSF 53. If that filter adds an ultraviolet light, it would also carry the NSF 55 standard. The reverse osmosis example from the previous paragraph would be a NSF 53/58 and most likely also add NSF 42.

The most common water filters purchased for home are NSF 42 and NSF 53. This is the most affordable option to obtain water that's treated under NSF 42 for taste and appearance, and under NSF 53 for 'some' health related contaminants.

From the NSF website, they define the two standards as follows:

NSF/ANSI Standard 42: Drinking Water Treatment Units - Aesthetic Effects

NSF/ANSI Standard 42 establishes the minimum requirements for the certification of Point of Use (POU) or Point of Entry (POE) filtration systems designed to reduce specific aesthetic or non-health-related contaminants (chlorine, taste, odor and particulates) that may be present in public or private drinking water.

The scope of NSF/ANSI 42 includes material safety, structural integrity and aesthetic, non-health-related contaminant reduction performance claims. The most common technology addressed by this standard is carbon filtration.

NSF/ANSI Standard 53: Drinking Water Treatment Units - Health Effects

NSF/ANSI Standard 53 establishes the minimum requirements for the certification of POU/POE filtration systems designed to reduce specific health-related contaminants, such as Cryptosporidium, Giardia, lead, volatile organic chemicals (VOCs) and MTBE (methyl tertiary-butyl ether), that may be present in public or private drinking water.

The scope of NSF/ANSI 53 includes material safety, structural integrity and health-related contaminant reduction performance claims. The most common technology addressed by this standard is carbon filtration.

Source: http://www.nsf.org/services/by-industry/water-wastewater/residential-water-treatment/residential-drinking-water-treatment-standards

8. Understanding NSF Standards and Protocols

NSF breaks down water filter standards and protocols in five general classifications. I like to label them in as Good, Better and Best.

A good filter is labeled NSF 42. Protocol 42 only concerns itself with the aesthetics of water: the look, smell, and taste. Generally, the two items a NSF 42 filter removes is chlorine (or chlorophyll) and particulates.

Removing chlorine will make water taste and smell better. Removing particulates (dirt and scale) gives water a crystal-clear appearance.

The most basic water filters are NSF 42 certified with prices starting around $20. If you see NSF 42 on the water filter packaging, you know it meets the NSF minimum for removing chlorine and dirt.

The NSF minimum for chlorine removal is 50%. If the packaging doesn't list how much chlorine it is removing (e.g. 97%) but still has the NSF logo, it could be either of these classes:

- Class I, a minimum of 75% chlorine reduction.
- Class II, 50% chlorine reduction.

This is why you want to purchase a filter that not only is NSF certified but also indicates how much chlorine is being removed.

Particulates are rated by the size of particulate the filter removes. They are listed as Class I through VI. Class I removes the smallest particulates, and Class VI removes the largest.

If the filter does not list which Particulate Class it is rated for and still has the NSF logo, it could be a Class VI filter which doesn't remove anything smaller than a grain of sand.

For mechanical filtration, the classes represent particle size ranges that are removed with a minimum 85% efficiency:

- Class VI, 50+ microns
- Class V, 30-50 microns - removes particulates no smaller than a grain of beach sand.
- Class IV, 15-30 microns - removes particulates no smaller than small grit.
- Class III, 5-15 microns - removes particulates that make water discolored and muddy.
- Class II, 1-5 microns
- Class I, ½ -1 micron - removes the smallest particulates including Cryptosporidium & Giardia Cysts.

If a filter is made from paper, string, or poly spun, it's only designed to remove rust and sediment from 5 to 40 micros

(Classes II through IV). However, carbon block filters remove 0.5 micro sized particulates. Therefore, a well designed filter has a carbon block core that is wrapped with paper or a poly spun material on the outside.

A better filter is a NSF 53 which removes health related contaminants. The best filter adds ultraviolet light to kill microorganisms.

The next section presents actual manufacturer specification sheets for water filters. You will learn how the NSF ratings are listed and what to look for on these real spec sheets.

9. How to Read a Water Filter Performance Data Sheet

When NSF approves a filter after it passes their certification process, NSF also determines how that information can be displayed on the product packaging and specification sheet.

Here's an example:

> *"System tested and certified by NSF international against NSF/ANSI standard 53 and NSF/ANSI standard 42 for the reduction claims specified on the performance data sheet."*

Unfortunately, there is no uniformity in how manufacturers display this information.

Below, you will see a few performance specification sheets and learn how to find the information you're looking for to determine if a filter is NSF certified and for which contaminants. You'll see some spec sheets with a lot of detail and some with very little.

The other tricky part of understanding NSF standards is that they work off an "A La Carte" type of system. You have to dig a bit deeper than just the logo and/or certification statement and locate the supporting chart and/or detailed list of contaminants that the unit claim refers to, commonly called the data performance sheet.

One products' data sheet may include a long list of contaminants while another might just include a few. Both can claim the same NSF certifications.

For instance, according to Brita, their standard replacement filter (Part# OB03) for their pitcher style of product is certified to NSF Standards 42 and 53 but when you look closer, the certification is for only 5 contaminants of the many contaminants under NSF 53.

Knowing how to interpret a performance sheet will aid you in selecting the correct filter for you and your family. Below are a few real examples of product data sheets and some hints on how to read them.

Example 1. Clean&Pure

Clean&Pure is a very popular filter that's sold on Home Shopping Network. Here are the things to pay attention to with their label.

The NSF logo appears. That indicates the unit has been approved. The text in the box next to the logo reads:

> *'Tested and certified by NSF against NSF/ANSI Standard 42 for the aesthetic reduction of chlorine. Particulate Class V.'*

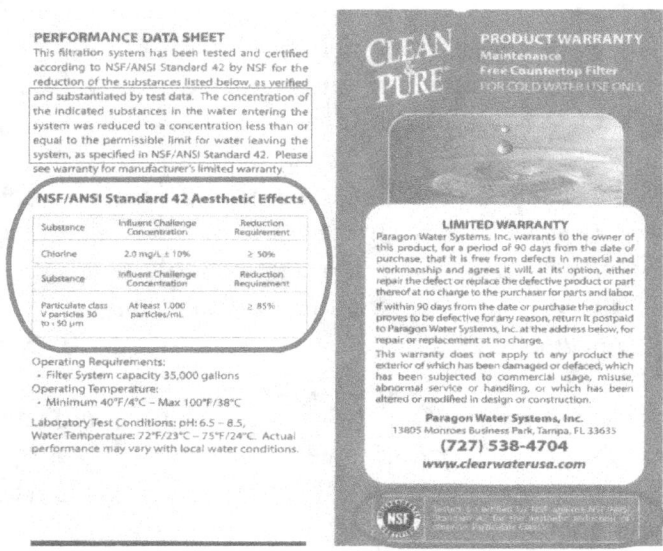

Here's the statement that explains why they are permitted to show the NSF logo.

> *'The concentration of the indicated substances in the water entering the unit was reduced to a concentration less than or equal to the permissible limit for water leaving the unit, as specified by NSF/ANSI Standard 42.'*

The table shows what substances are being removed on the left, and the NSF Standard 42 minimal permissible limit (greater than 50% removal for chlorine – greater than 85% removal for particulates).

For chlorine, we don't know the exact amount of reduction this filter achieves. We just know that at least 50% of the chlorine is reduced. If you want a unit that removed over 90% of the chlorine, this probably wouldn't be the one to buy.

This filter removes Class V particulates which is the largest size allowed by NSF. If you wanted a unit that removes the smallest particulate size (Class I), this would not be the filter to get.

You can easily find a NSF 42 filter that removes over 90% of chlorine and over 90% of Class I particulates for under $30. Or, you can pay nearly the same money for a filter that doesn't make a reduction level claim other than that it meets the minimum NSF standard.

Knowing what to look for in a filter can be determined by learning to read the product performance sheet.

Example 2. WaterChef

Here is another NSF/ANSI 42 filter that also includes NSF/ANSI 53 certification.

It contains the NSF logo and a description that reads…

> *'System tested and certified by NSF International against NSF/ANSI Standard 42 for the reduction of Chloramine, Chlorine tastes and odor, and nominal particulate Class I…*

'...and NSF/ANSI Standard 53 for the reduction of Cysts, Lead, VOC and MTBE'

The NSF/ANSI Standard 42 (Aesthetic Effects) specifications will always be a small table of specs because it only consists of chlorine and/or chloramine, and particulate.

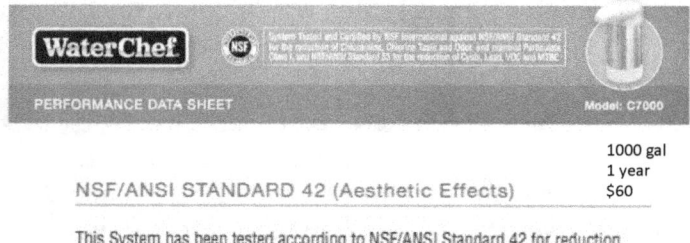

Unlike the Clean&Pure table from the last example, the WaterChef NSF 42 table adds a column that list the Actual % Reduction – chlorine 93.1%; chloramine 93.1%; particulate >99%.

NSF approved WaterChef for their 93.1% reduction of chlorine and chloramine and its >99% reduction of particulate, unlike Clean&Pure which was NSF approved for only meeting NSF minimum standards.

The WaterChef clearly lists the level of reduction the filter achieves for chlorine/chloramine and particulates. And, it's removing the smallest group of particulates, Class I, where the Clean&Pure was only approved to reduce Class V, a much larger sized piece of dirt.

The NSF/ANSI Standard 53 (Health Effects) specifications table will be as large as there are contaminants the filter is designed to reduce. Some NSF 53 filters only remove a few health related contaminants while other filters remove dozens of contaminants.

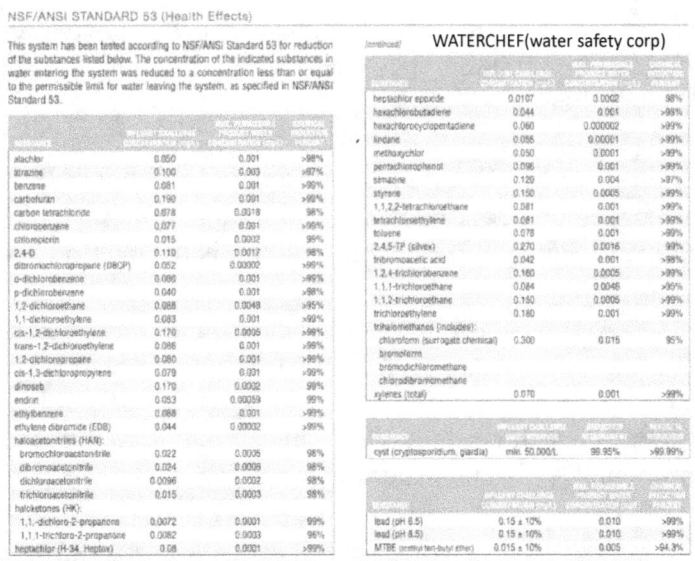

The WaterChef folks designed their label with three separate tables to highlight the different groups of NSF 53 contaminants they reduce. As I mentioned earlier, there is no standard method to display this information on performance data sheets, which sometimes makes it difficult to compare one filter to another without careful inspection of the labels.

The first table lists a bunch of items in alphabetical order from Alachlor to Xylenes. The next table shows Cyst, and the last table shows Lead and MTBE. The most important number is in the far right column: Chemical or Actual Reduction %.

Example 3: Brita

To demonstrate the various looks of a water filter spec sheet, below is one for a NSF 42/53 filter made by Brita. There are a few things different on this spec sheet (Brita) than the one above (WaterChef).

Brita list the NSF 53 information first and puts all their NSF 53 substances in one box. Brita adds a lot more columns in their chart (the 'Percent Reduction' column is the one to find).

Brita lists VOC as the last item on the chart. VOCs are a group of volatile organic compounds and the filter must reduce each of those compounds to a certain level to be approved for the entire VOC family of compounds. You can't 'A-La-Cart' the VOC compounds. It's all or nothing with VOCs.

(I don't expect that you can read the chart with its small print. I wanted to show how different it looks from the others).

BRITA® FAUCET FILTRATION SYSTEM
MODEL FF-100 WITH FILTER FR-200

SUBSTANCE	REDUCTION						U.S. EPA Level[*]/ NSF Max. Permissible Product Water Concentration	HEALTH CANADA GUIDELINE	TESTING PARAMETERS		
	Influent Challenge Concentration		Filter Effluent		Percent Reduction				Alkalinity ppm CaCO₃	Temp. (°C)	pH
	Actual	NSF Target	Average	Maximum	Average	Minimum					
NSF/ANSI Standard 53 – Health Effects											
Asbestos	90⁶	10–100⁶	<0.17⁶	<0.17⁶	>99%	>99%	7/99%⁶	N.A.	N.A.	19	7.4
Lead	150 ppb	150±15 ppb	<1 ppb	<1 ppb	>99.3%	>99.3%	15 ppb/10 ppb	10 ppb¹	18	21	6.5
Lead	150 ppb	150±15 ppb	<1 ppb	<1 ppb	>99.3%	>99.3%	15 ppb/10 ppb	10 ppb²	100	20	8.4
Cyster	92,000⁷	≥50,000⁷	<1⁷	<1⁷	>99.99%	>99.99%	99.9%/99.95%⁷	N.A.	N.A.	20	7.9
Alachlor	40 ppb	40±4 ppb	<1 ppb	<1 ppb	>97.5%	>97.5%	2 ppb	N.A.	N.A.	20	7.2
Atrazine	10 ppb	9±0.9 ppb	<0.5 ppb	<0.5 ppb	>95%	>95%	3 ppb	5 ppb²	21	7.4
Benzene	15 ppb	15±1.5 ppb	<0.5 ppb	<0.5 ppb	>96.6%	>96.6%	5 ppb	5 ppb²	21	7.6
Carbofuran	77 ppb	80±8 ppb	<1 ppb	<1 ppb	>98.7%	>98.7%	40 ppb	90 ppb³	N.A.	20	7.4
Carbon tetrachloride	14 ppb	15±1.5 ppb	<0.5 ppb	<0.5 ppb	>96.5%	>96.5%	5 ppb	2 ppb²	N.A.	20	7.4
Chlordane	42 ppb	40±4 ppb	0.4 ppb	2.8 ppb	98.9%	95.2%	2 ppb	N.A.	N.A.	20	7.3
Chlorobenzene	2.0 ppm	2.0±0.2 ppm	0.002 ppm	0.019 ppm	99.9%	99%	0.1 ppm	0.06 ppm²	N.A.	20	7.3
o-Dichlorobenzene	1.9 ppm	1.8±0.18 ppm	<0.0005 ppm	<0.0005 ppm	>99.9%	>99.9%	0.6 ppm	0.2 ppm²	N.A.	21	7.4
2,4-D	210 ppb	210±21 ppb	0.1 ppb	0.2 ppb	99.9%	99.9%	70 ppb	100 ppb²	N.A.	20	7.4
Endrin	6.6 ppb	6±0.6 ppb	<0.2 ppb	<0.2 ppb	>97%	>97%	2 ppb	N.A.	N.A.	21	7.6
Ethylbenzene	2.2 ppm	2.1±0.21 ppm	0.0007 ppm	0.0031 ppm	99.9%	99.8%	0.7 ppm	≤0.0024 ppm²	N.A.	21	7.4
Lindane	2.0 ppb	2±0.2 ppb	<0.02 ppb	<0.02 ppb	>99%	>99%	0.2 ppb	N.A.	N.A.	20	7.4
Methoxychlor	120 ppb	120±12 ppb	0.4 ppb	0.7 ppb	99.7%	99.3%	40 ppb	N.A.	N.A.	22	7.4
Simazine	11 ppb	12±1.2 ppb	1.4 ppb	4 ppb	87%	63%	4 ppb	10 ppb²	N.A.	20	7.6
Styrene	1.9 ppm	2.0±0.2 ppm	<0.0005 ppm	<0.0005 ppm	>99.9%	>99.9%	0.1 ppm	N.A.	N.A.	20	7.2
Tetrachloroethylene	16 ppb	15±1.5 ppb	<0.5 ppb	<0.5 ppb	>96.9%	>96.4%	5 ppb	30 ppb²	N.A.	20	7.4
Toluene	3.1 ppm	3.0±0.3 ppm	<0.0005 ppm	<0.0005 ppm	>99.9%	>99.9%	1 ppm	≤0.024 ppm²	N.A.	20	7.2
Toxaphene	16 ppb	15±1.5 ppb	<1 ppb	<1 ppb	>93.6%	>93.6%	3 ppb	N.A.	N.A.	20	7.3
Trichloroethylene	320 ppb	300±30 ppb	<0.5 ppb	<0.5 ppb	>99.8%	>99.8%	5 ppb	5 ppb²	N.A.	21	7.4
TTHM	390 ppb	450±90 ppb	4.6 ppb	22 ppb	98.7%	94.3%	80 ppb	100 ppb	N.A.	21	7.5
Turbidity	11 NTU⁷	11±1 NTU⁷	0.1 NTU⁷	0.1 NTU⁷	99%	99%	0.3–1.0 NTU⁷/0.5 NTU⁷	0.1–1 NTU⁷	N.A.	20	7.4
VOC	290 ppb	330±30 ppb	0.6 ppb	1.3 ppb	99.7%	99.5%	N.A.	N.A.	N.A.	20	7.3
NSF/ANSI Standard 42 – Aesthetic Effects											
Chlorine taste and odor	2.0 ppm	2.0±0.2 ppm	0.05 ppm	0.05 ppm	97.3%	97.4%	N.A./50%³	N.A.	N.A.	20	7.4
Particulate (Class L 0.5–1.0 μm)	5,700,000⁷	≥10,000⁷	21,000⁷	27,000⁷	99.7%	99.6%	N.A./85%⁷	N.A.	N.A.	20	7.3

100 gal
3-4 month
$20

The WaterChef choose to list the VOCs individually by their chemical name, which is why you don't see a listing named VOC on the WaterChef chart. It makes their chart look like its removing more compounds when they list the VOC compounds individually as opposed to just listing VOC as a Brita does.

For NSF 42, Brita list the chlorine and particulate data on the bottom of the chart. Brita does not list Chloramine but WaterChef does. They both are removing Class I size particulates.

Brita removes more chlorine and particulate than WaterChef (97.5 vs 93.1%). However, the WaterChef listing only represents that the filter was tested at NSF to remove at least 93.1%. Because it passed at 93.1% it can be listed on the spec sheet. But, WaterChef may have tested to that same level as Brita (97.5%) but only claims to remove the 93.1% they list on their spec sheet.

In other words, filters are only permitted to list what they request NSF to approve them for. If NSF certifies that amount of reduction has been met, that number can be listed on the performance data sheet. If NSF determines through their test that the reduction exceeded that number, they'd never tell the manufacturer. As far as NSF is concerned, the filter achieved the level reduction the manufacturer claimed it would.

On the other hand, if the filter failed to meet that number, NSF will consider that test a failure and the manufacturer would have to reengineer their unit or submit a lower level of reduction for NSF approval.

Or, in the case of Clean&Pure, they claim to only meet the NSF minimum standard in order to get approval without providing an actual reduction claim. As long as NSF determines the Clean&Pure meets their minimum standard, the unit becomes NSF certified. For example, they meet the

50% minimum reduction for chlorine, but they can't later claim they remove 60% of chlorine without verification from NSF.

Comparing spec sheets is not as easy as it should be, but when you know what you're looking for, you can find what you're looking for on the performance data sheet. Just don't expect every manufacturer to stick with a standard format for presenting the information.

The other information you want to look for on the product packaging is:
- The number of gallons the filter is rated for
- The number of months the filter is rated for

Be aware that no filter unit has a meter to tell you how many gallons has gone through the filter but some of the better filters will add a filter indicator to let you know when it's time to be replaced.

Beware that the flow rate of water coming out of the filter will slow down when the filter is getting old and becomes clogged with contaminants. Depending on how much material the filter has blocked determines how long the filter will last. Extreme 'dirty' water may render a filter useless before it reaches the listed limit.

This is an issue with the very small filters found on faucet mounted and refrigerator filters. When new, the water comes out fast. As it ages and contaminants start to plug up the filter the water begins to slow down considerably.

10. Top Brands of Water Filters

I would argue that the top brands of home water filters are any brand that is certified with NSF. When a unit has the NSF logo on it you can be assured that it has gone through a thorough independent test from a legitimate 3rd party lab that confirms that the product claims made by the manufacturer was achieved, and possibly exceeded.

That is not to say that there are filter manufacturers who don't meet those same standards. Several companies claim that they meet NSF standards but cannot post the NSF logo on their product because NSF didn't test it. It's up to your level of trust to accept their data as being honest and true.

This was presented earlier in this publication but it's worth repeating again here:

Here is a real example of a filter manufacturer performance specification who claims to meet NSF standards but did not have their unit certified with NSF…

> *The Clear2O ® ADVANCED CWF500 series filter has been independently tested on over 200 contaminants to achieve water industry standards NSF/ANSI 42 and NSF/ANSI 53 for reduction of Chlorine, Heavy Metals, Cysts, VOC, & Other contaminants. The Clear2O® ADVANCED filter system surpasses NSF/ANSI 53 and NSF/ANSI 401 test standards for removal of*

Herbicides, Pesticides, Pharmaceuticals, Industrial Wastes, and PFOA's (Perfluorooctanoic Acids), man-made chemicals used in various manufacturing processes, and has been shown to be a health concern as it has been shown to be widely present in the environment and remain in the human body for long periods of time.

This unit is not NSF certified. However, they claim to have surpassed NSF test standards. It's up to you to believe that claim or not. If the Clear2O unit sent their unit to NSF to obtain NSF certification, there would be no doubt that their claims are verified.

I personally have a favorite certified filter that I've been using for years. I purposely will not list it in this publication. I don't want to offer any bias to any manufacturer in this publication. My purpose for writing this document is to give you all the information you need to make an informed decision on the water filter you select.

However, if you email me with 'What's your favorite water filter?' in the subject line, I'll be happy to respond with my favorite choice.

DWD@dirtywaterdude.com

NSF listing for certified filters:
http://info.nsf.org/Certified/PwsComponents

Conclusion

I believe water filters will soon become mandatory based on the increased prevalence of homes identified as being served by water systems that have violations in their water treatment process. You don't have to wait until you receive a 'boil water alert' or find that your city has an outbreak as bad as Flint or Toledo. You can take action now.

A certified water filter, when used properly, will protect you from many harmful contaminants – known and unknown – every day. Most times, a home filter will far exceed bottled water in the removal of contaminants. And, at $1 for a bottle of water, that same $1 will buy you 500 bottles of tap water, on average.

I fill a thermos with filtered water from home before I leave the house every day to make sure I have clean, safe water with me at all times. And, when it comes home empty at the end of the day, I know I've consumed the recommended daily amount of water the experts suggest.

A good water filter is well worth the investment. Just remember, it's critical to replace the filter cartridges according to the manufacturer's recommendation in order for your filter unit to consistently reduce contaminants as the specifications indicate.

On average, you will pay about $100 a year in replacement filter cartridges to keep your filter unit performing perfectly everyday of your life. For less than a nickel a day, you can drink a virtual endless supply of clean safe water right from your home.

If you don't use a water filter, you become the water filter.

Stefan Roots
The Dirty Water Dude

> Email: dwd@DirtyWaterDude.com
> Web Site: DirtyWaterDude.com
> Twitter: @DirtyWaterDude
> Podcast: Dirty Water Dude on iTunes and other podcast apps